Maintaining Balance with a Power of Attorney

Principal (Book 1 of 2)

EO Writes

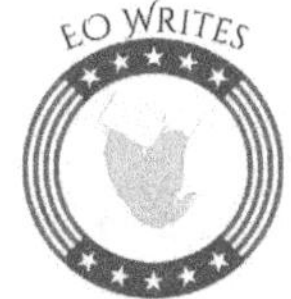

EO Writes lizzy@eowrites.com

Book cover designed by EO Writes. Photos from my own personal collection.

Contents

Dedication

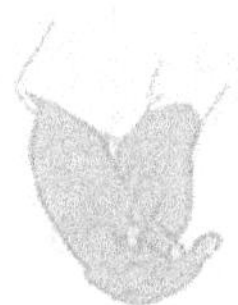

This book was a labor of love. I dedicated this book to those who walked alongside me on the path I took with my parents in their last year. First of all, I could not have done it without God. Secondly, I learned that none of us accomplish things alone. We are not a team of one, but many.

Thirdly, God's will was for me to be my parent's Power of Attorney, and he equipped me for that role. The position led to a heart change and restoration in my relationship with them. As a result, I had peace when they passed on.

Introduction

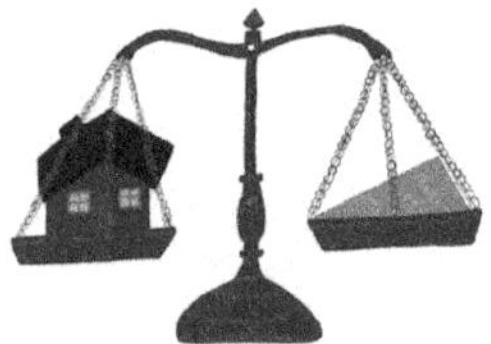

The content in this book is for informational purposes only. I am not a lawyer and am not giving legal advice. Consult with a lawyer if you have questions regarding obtaining a Power of Attorney or the use of one. This book was written based on my experience as a Power of Attorney for my parents.

My Parent's Story

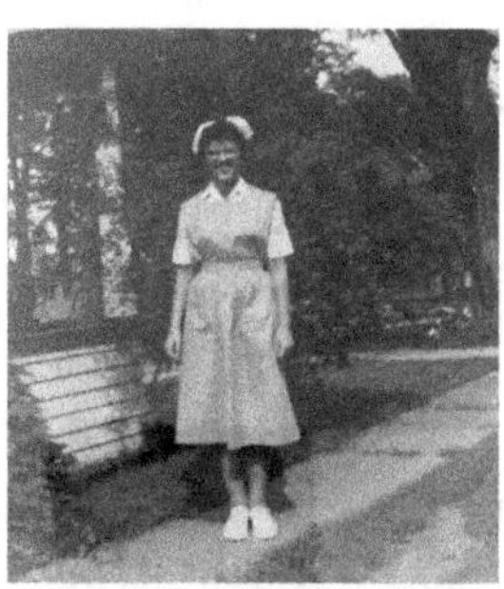

Mom, as a Candy Striper

How my parents met has always fascinated me. Dad was admitted to the hospital for further testing due to migraine headaches, mom was a Candy Striper. One day, she went by his room and caught his eye. Every time she went by his room, he would sing to her Beautiful Brown Eyes.

Later, he had caught her heart as well! They got married, had 5 kids, 15 grandchildren, and two great grandchildren. Fifty-eight years later and they were still in love. Don't get me wrong, they had their spouts, but they stood the test of time.

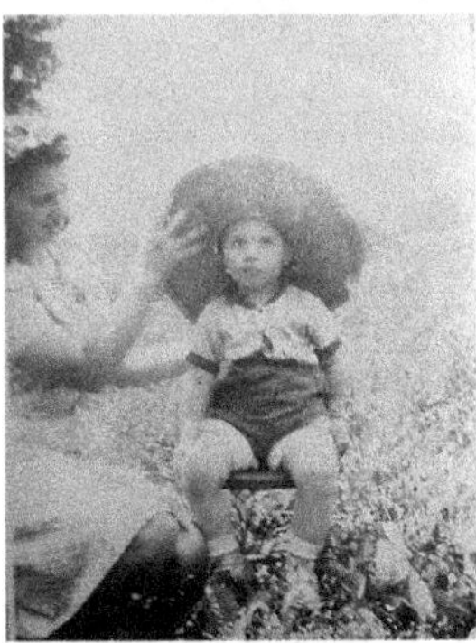

Dad

My dad was a man of wits, he loved to clown around. He had a knack for making me laugh. He was a hard worker, a high-scoring bowler, and a praiser. I don't recall him ever complaining about his job.

He just did what he needed to do for his family. He was a God-fearing man that understood the vow he had made to my mom and to his family. Many a Saturday morning, I would find my dad sitting in his recliner, hymnals in hand, singing to the Lord. He was always singing. I guess that is why, to this day, I prefer my hymnal.

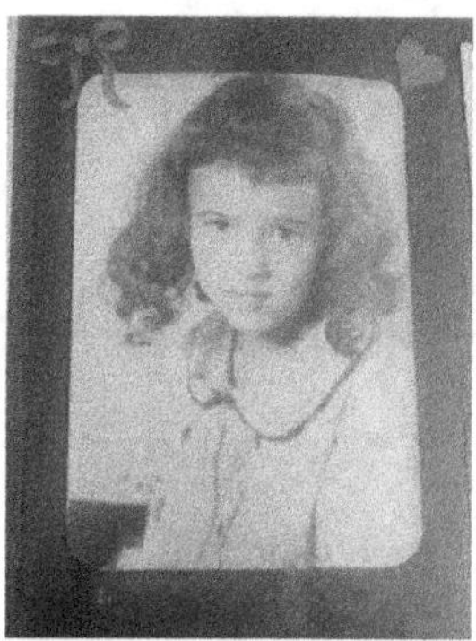

Mom

My mom was a hard worker and loved to make crafts. She was always busy with her hands. If she wasn't baking, you could find her scrapbooking, making bookmarks, cards. When I was young, she made clothes for my Barbie's.

She also enjoyed cross stitching and crocheting. She made my daughter a Raggedy Ann and Andy doll, which she still has to this day. My mom loved to share what she created with others, whether it was dish rags, hand towels and/or cookies at Christmas.

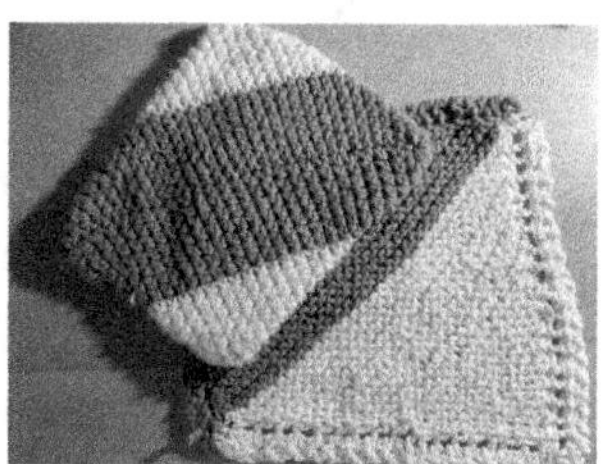

A dish rag and hot mitt she made.

My Daddy

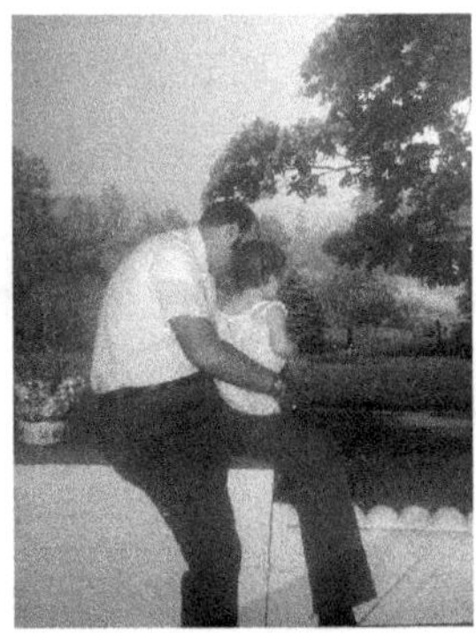

My daddy and I.

My Daddy

Was a man of great strength and wit.

He knew the value of hard work & he wasn't one to quit.

He believed in God and his dear Son and sang of the victories he had already won.

He worked ever so faithfully with his hands and kept his wedding vows to the end.

A father, A husband, A friend these are just a few titles given to men.

But when it comes to one's story, may it be

"one who was faithful" – "one who gave his all to Him.

FAITHFUL

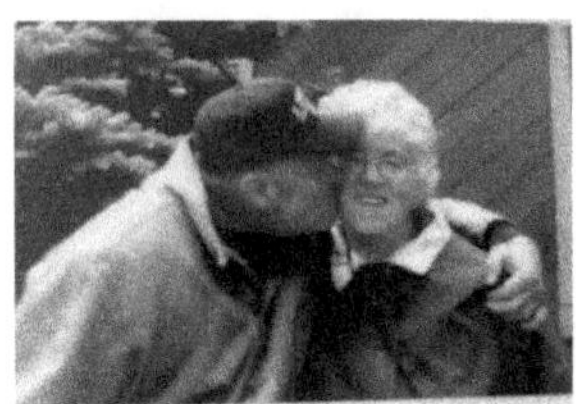

My parents

My parents believed in hard work. Us kids grew up helping dad with the planting and harvesting of crops: such as corn, peas, cucumbers, squash, etc. My mom was always hard at work baking cinnamon rolls, canning jelly, picking berries, etc. My dad loved to work with his hands. He built me a huge wooden doll house.

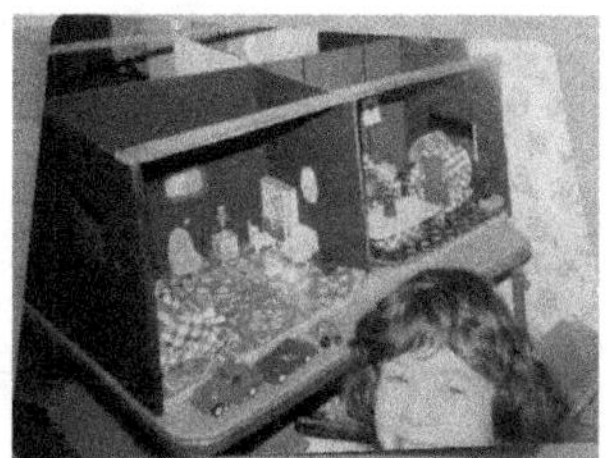
Barbie doll house

He even made a wooden box for my kitty "Toby," which we buried back in the woods behind the house.

One of my fondest memories is of a doll bed that he made me. In, his later years, he restored it to its former glory and made me a much needed stable for my nativity set.

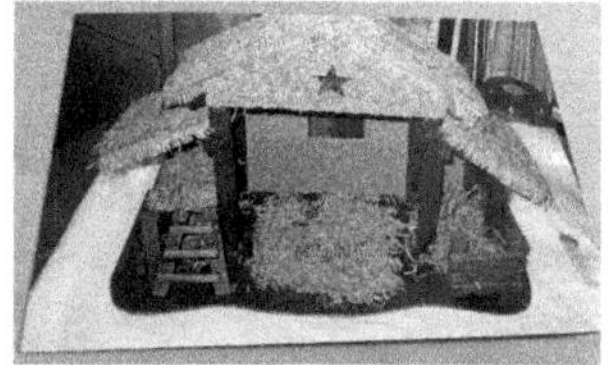
Stable

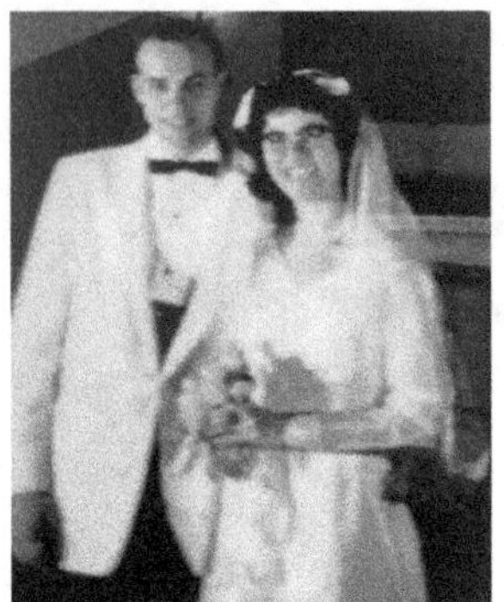

October 17, 1959

Traditional Wedding Vows

"I take you, to be my wedded wife/ husband, to have and to hold from this day forward, for better, for worse, for richer, for poorer, in sickness and in health, to love and to cherish till death do us part, according to God's holy ordinance; and thereto I pledge thee my faith [or] pledge myself to you."

What is a Power of Attorney?

A Power of Attorney is a legal document which gives another authority over one's financial matters. The person who you designate to be custodian of the Power of Attorney for you is your Agent.

Prayerfully consider who you want to assist you in your financial matters. They will be your voice; however, I assure you are not voiceless. They only have the power you give them. You can choose limited to broad powers. You can terminate the Power of Attorney for any reason.

An Agent cannot make healthcare decisions for you. You will need a Health Care Proxy to do that.

Power of Attorney, How Did I Acquire It?

It all started when my dad was coming home from a grocery trip. He lost his balance and fell down the stairs leading to their apartment downstairs. A neighbor near the stairs heard the commotion and came out to see what was going on. He cautioned my dad not to move and called for an ambulance after informing my mom of the situation. Due to the complexity of the break in his neck, he was transferred to a hospital outside of our area.

My mom spent many long hours visiting with my dad and restless nights. Obviously, the stress of the situation was getting to her. While my dad was in the hospital, my mom fell into a weakened state and admitted herself.

The stress of the situation aggravated her cancer symptoms. Hospice advised me of the gravity of the situation. Calls were made to siblings as mom's oxygen level depleted.

She looked as though she was at death's door. We thought at one point she would be gone in the night. But as dad recovered, so did mom. During one of my visits with my dad, his Hospice Case worker informed me that he had discussed with her that the bank was no longer accepting his checks due to illegible handwriting, caused by nerve damage from the fall.

Hospice Case worker suggested that I talk to him about becoming his Power of Attorney. I talked to my dad about it, to which he replied, "You have a good head on your shoulders." So right then and there, with the oversight of a Nurse and a Notary we did the paperwork designating me as his Power of Attorney. Before his release, their Hospice Caseworker stressed that he really shouldn't go back to that apartment. It was too risky with his balance issues and all.

They suggested that it was time to consider a nursing home for my parents to which my parents agreed, hesitantly. My mom was beside herself when I admitted her. Not long after, with the counsel of the Financial Advisor, mom agreed to designate me as her Power of Attorney as well.

My parents lived in the nursing home for about a year. My dad died in June and my mom died shortly after in August. I liken my parent's life to two eagles. Eagles love to do tricks in the sky. Sometimes a pair of eagles will lock their claws and spiral down thousands of feet. Before my parents passed, God said to me as they were in life so they will be in death.

> ...in their death they were not divided; They were swifter than eagles, they were stronger than lions.
>
> 2 Samuel 1:23b

My parent's devotion to one another until death is a stark reminder of God's devotion to us, His bride. They left an example for all of us.

God always has more in store when he calls us to do something. The Power of Attorney wasn't just for my parents but for me as well. As roles were reversed, I saw the child in my parents and whatever animosity that was there between us was turned to forgiveness and restoration, especially between my mom and me. When my job was complete, I had peace in my heart that I made amends with my parents.

How is it Obtained?

There are different ways you can obtain one:

1. A Law Firm

2. Hospital

3. Nursing Home

4. Through forms online

My father's Hospice Case Worker informed me that I could get a Power of Attorney form from the hospital, and that a Notary there would need to oversee us signing it. The Notary and a Nurse oversaw the signing. The form was called a New York Durable (Statutory) Power of Attorney Short Form, which gave me the power to facilitate my father's financial matters.

The Power of Attorney gave me the legal right to speak to others on his behalf regarding these matters. I also had a say over his medical matters due to being his health proxy. I obtained a Power of Attorney form for my mother through the Financial Advisor at the nursing home, who happened to be a Notary.

She witnessed us signing it and then notarized it. I do believe all nursing homes have a Notary present.

The form that I filled out with both of my parents was called a New York Durable (Statutory) Power of Attorney Short Form. You can choose limited to broad powers.

This gave me the power to oversee my parents' financial matters. To speak on their behalf in these matters. You can also go to the link below and print out a Power of Attorney form, according to the state you live in.

Article Title Power of Attorney (POA) Forms (11) URL https://eforms.com/power-of-attorney/

Website title forms/Date accessed January 20, 2026

Notary

You will both need to sign this before a witness and a Notary. The one you have designated as your Agent will have to present a copy of the Power of Attorney document that you both signed to all the financial institutions you are associated with. Your Agent cannot make any changes without this document.

The Power the Agent Yields

To recap, the one you have designated as your Agent has a say over your financial matters, but that doesn't mean you are without a voice. Be sure to meet with them often to discuss how you want your affairs handled once this is in place.

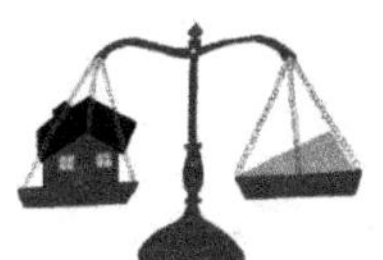

Important Information For Your Agent

Birth Date:

Social Security #

Life Insurance:

Life Insurance: policy #

Bank

Checking Account #'

Bill Account #"s

Funeral Home

The Agent's Responsibilities

They will assist you in your financial matters. They will need your life insurance policy number, birth date, social security number, and bills. My parents were in the nursing home during my time as their Agent, so I had their mail forwarded to my address, which made it easier to pay their bills in a timely matter.

They will need to know the name of the bank that holds your account. I added my name to their account on the advice of an Associate from their bank. They will need to show the bank the Power of Attorney document to be able to do this.

Can a Power of Attorney Be Revoked?

You can revoke your Power of Attorney for any reason as long as you are of sound mind. Print out a Power of Attorney Revocation Form (Cancel a POA) from the link on this page.

Instituting this form will cancel and void the previous Power of Attorney document. You will need to sign this before a witness and a Notary.

The Power of Attorney is canceled and immediately terminated upon signature. You will need to send this form to your Agent via *certified mail* and to all individuals, agencies, and institutions you are associated with. If they continue, it is a criminal act.

Power of Attorney (POA) Forms (11) URL https://eforms.com/power-of-attorney/

Website title forms/Date accessed January 20, 2026

Other than revoking the Power of Attorney, the Power of Attorney ends at your death.

TEMPLATES

These are for your personal use. Make as many copies as needed.

Inventory

To Do List

Notes

Contacts

Appointments

Journal

Journal

Journal

Journal

Journal

Journal

Journal

Journal

Journal

In Conclusion

I leave you with this final word. I hope this book has helped you understand what a Power of Attorney is, your rights and how having one can help alleviate some responsibility.

God called me to be an Agent for my father; however, I did not anticipate doing it for both my parents. I was my parents' Agent and Health Proxy for a year and learned a lot in that time. I am grateful that I oversaw my parent's care in their last year.

Remember now thy Creator in the days of thy youth, while the evil days come not, nor the years draw nigh, when thou shalt say, I have no pleasure in them.

Ecclesiastes 12:1

Let us hear the conclusion of the whole matter: fear God and keep his commandments:for this is the whole duty of man.

Ecclesiastes 12:2

Glossary

The Power of Attorney is a legal document that gives the Agent a say over the principal's financial matters.

POA is another name for The Power of Attorney.

Principal is the one whom the Agent serves.

The Agent is the one who serves the Principal.

The beneficiary is the individual the insurance pays out to in case of the policyholder's death.

Contingent a beneficiary child of the policyholder if the beneficiary is no longer living.

Policyholder is the one who holds the insurance. (Principal)

Care Plan meetings are requested by either the resident (of a nursing home) or the Agent if there needs to be an evaluation of care.

Trust Fund (aka Personal Accounts) A resident (of a nursing home) can have money allocated to a personal account for them to use. A resident can use these funds for their bills such as cable, phone, etc. They will let you know when they get low.

Hospice is for people who are nearing the end of life. Hospice provides services through a team of healthcare professionals who maximize comfort for a person who is terminally ill by reducing pain and addressing physical, psychological, social, and spiritual needs.

Financial Institution A business that deals with financial and monetary transactions (For example: banks, insurance companies, investment dealers, and brokerage firms)

About the Author

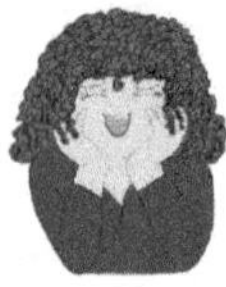

EO Writes has been married for 28 years. She and her husband enjoy riding their Harley throughout the United States. Her passion is sharing God's love through her art and writing. She hopes to get her children's book, Luna Goes Exploring published in 2026.

"Never judge a book by its cover. What you find inside the pages might surprise you."

Note from the Author:

"A word fitly spoken is like apples of gold in pictures of silver.

Proverbs 25:11

If you have enjoyed this book, would you consider leaving a review on Amazon? Thank you!

Also by EO Writes

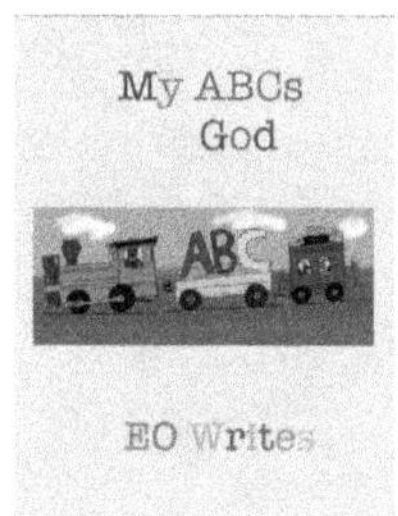

My ABCs & God

A great way to introduce your child or student to the alphabet, to an unfamiliar word, a unique character, a Bible verse, and a coloring page. This is a great addition to a Kindergarten curriculum for a homeschool parent or a Christian school.

https://www.amazon.com/dp/B0GCTYGPQM

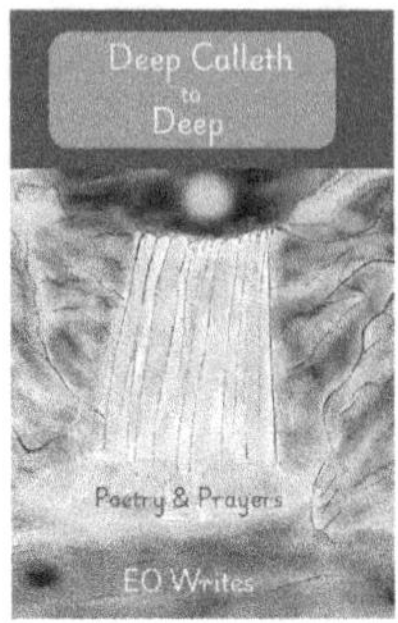

Deep Calleth to Deep

A collection of poetry and prayers that come from my heart to yours. I hope you will find encouragement on your journey with God through my words.

https://www.amazon.com/dp/B0FX594GMN

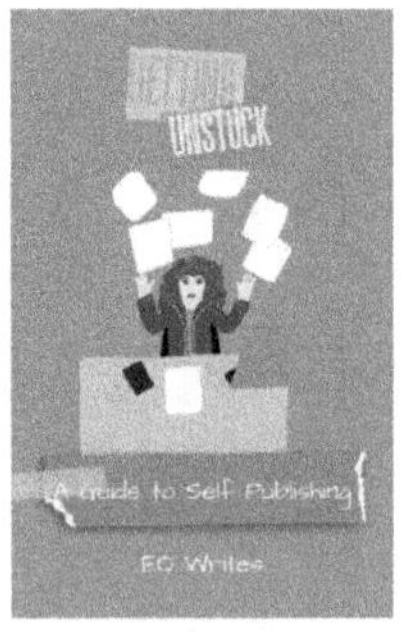

Getting Unstuck: A Guide to Self Publishing

Is it your dream to be a self publisher?

Do you have questions on the process, such as the steps for writing your story, the cost of self publishing, how to create illustrations for your book, editing and formatting? Let Getting Unstuck: A Guide to Self Publishing be your guide on your journey to self publishing.

https://www.amazon.com/dp/B0FC33TF94

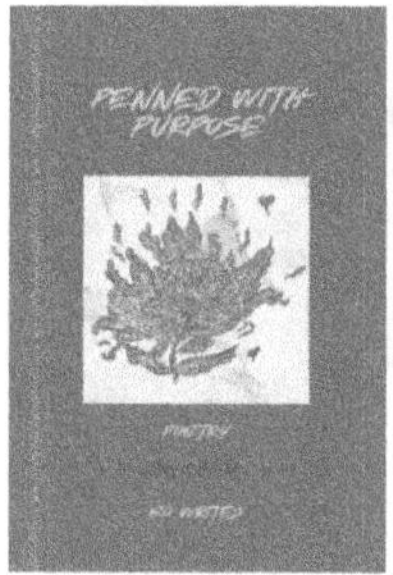

Penned with Purpose

An accumulation of poems that I have written over a couple of decades.

https://www.amazon.com/dp/B0DPMKGTRW

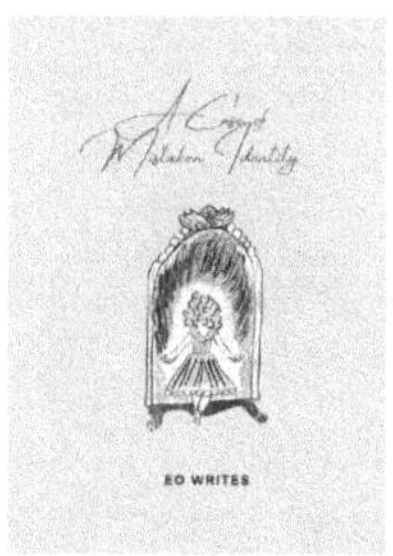

A Case of Mistaken Identity

Have you ever felt like the entire world was against you? In a case of mistaken identity, Sadie feels this way as a court trial challenges her deserving of a happy ending. Participants from both sides of the political spectrum are testifying in this pivotal court case, as her reputation is at stake. Those against her are claiming she is undeserving of her purpose. Is the Judge going to clear her of all accusations and give her a chance to start anew? In order to move forward with confidence, she needs to redeem her past.

https://www.amazon.com//dp/B0DPG25JLN

www.ingramcontent.com/pod-product-compliance
Lightning Source LLC
LaVergne TN
LVHW010945110826
845149LV00013B/2758

* 9 7 9 8 9 9 0 4 5 9 9 9 1 *